THE CIRCULATORY SYSTEM

By Autumn Leigh

Gareth Stevens
Publishing

Please visit our website, www.garethstevens.com. For a free color catalog of all our high-quality books, call toll free 1-800-542-2595 or fax 1-877-542-2596.

Library of Congress Cataloging-in-Publication Data

Leigh, Autumn, 1971-
The circulatory system / Autumn Leigh.
    p. cm. — (The human body)
Includes bibliographical references and index.
ISBN 978-1-4339-6579-1 (pbk.)
ISBN 978-1-4339-6580-7 (6-pack)
ISBN 978-1-4339-6577-7 (library binding)
1. Cardiovascular system—Juvenile literature. I. Title.
QP103.L45 2012
612.1—dc23
                                        2011020150

First Edition

Published in 2012 by
Gareth Stevens Publishing
111 East 14th Street, Suite 349
New York, NY 10003

Designer: Daniel Hosek
Editor: Greg Roza

Photo credits: Cover, p. 1 artpartner-images/Photographer's Choice/Getty Images; all backgrounds, pp. 5 (all images), 7 (heart), 9, 11 (all images), 13 (circulatory system), 15 (human body), 17 (all images), 18, 25 (blood pressure), 28–29 Shutterstock.com; pp. 7 (boy), 15 (kidney), 19, 25 (stents) Thinkstock.com; p. 13 (artery cross section) De Agostini Picture Library/Getty Images; p. 21 (white blood cells) Dr. Donald Fawcett & E. Shelton/Visuals Unlimited/Getty Images; p. 21 (platelets) Steve Gschmeissner/Science Photo Library/Getty Images; p. 22 Purestock/Getty Images; p. 27 Dr. Stanley Flegler/ Visuals Unlimited/Getty Images.

Printed in the United States of America

CPSIA compliance information: Batch #CW12GS: For further information contact Gareth Stevens, New York, New York at 1-800-542-2595.

Contents

Words in the glossary appear in **bold** type
the first time they are used in the text.

Around and Around We Go

Blood is constantly circulating, or moving, throughout the human body, pushed through blood vessels by the pumping of the heart. Together, the blood, blood vessels, and heart make up the circulatory system. Without a circulatory system, our bodies wouldn't be able to function the way they do. In fact, we wouldn't be able to live.

The circulatory system has two main jobs within the human body. First, it's responsible for transporting **nutrients**, water, oxygen, and chemicals to organs and tissues all over our bodies. It delivers all the things a body needs to function properly. Second, it transports waste products, such as carbon dioxide, to locations where they can be eliminated, or removed, from the body.

IN THE FLESH

The word "cardiac" means "having to do with the heart."

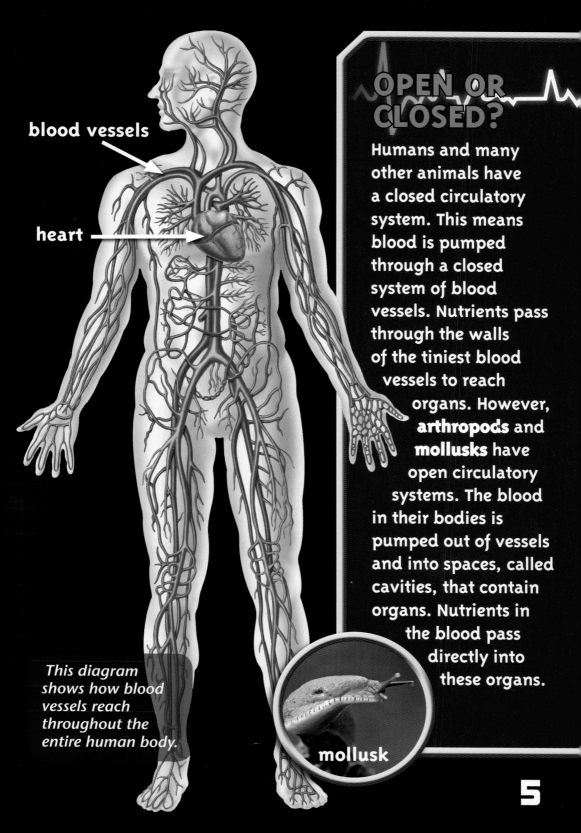

blood vessels

heart

This diagram shows how blood vessels reach throughout the entire human body.

mollusk

OPEN OR CLOSED?

Humans and many other animals have a closed circulatory system. This means blood is pumped through a closed system of blood vessels. Nutrients pass through the walls of the tiniest blood vessels to reach organs. However, **arthropods** and **mollusks** have open circulatory systems. The blood in their bodies is pumped out of vessels and into spaces, called cavities, that contain organs. Nutrients in the blood pass directly into these organs.

The Heart

You might consider your heart the motor of your circulatory system. It makes sure blood is always moving through the blood vessels, even when you're asleep. This ensures that the circulatory system continuously supplies our cells and organs with fresh nutrients and oxygen while removing waste products.

Your heart is about the size of your fist. It's located in the middle of your chest, between your lungs and slightly to the left side of your body. The rib cage keeps it safe. The heart is a special kind of muscle. We don't have to think about moving our heart as we do muscles such as those in our arms and legs. The heart keeps moving on its own.

IN THE FLESH

Every day, approximately 2,000 gallons (7,571 l) of blood pass through the human heart.

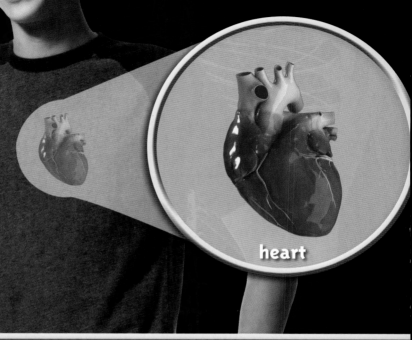

The heart is sometimes called the cardiac muscle.

heart

THE BEAT GOES ON

When you put your hand up to your chest, you can feel your heart beating. What you're feeling is your heart expanding (getting bigger) and contracting (getting smaller) very quickly. This movement is what keeps your blood flowing. A single heartbeat lasts about 0.8 second. The average human heart beats about 75 times a minute, 100,000 times a day, and 40 million times a year. It can beat 3 billion times in a lifetime.

The human heart is a pump. Actually, it's two pumps. The heart has four chambers arranged on two sides. The upper and lower chambers on each side form a pump. Each upper chamber is called an atrium. Each lower, larger chamber is called a ventricle.

The atrium on the right side of the heart receives blood from the body. Blood passes from the atrium into the right ventricle and is pumped to the lungs. The left atrium receives blood from the lungs, and the left ventricle pumps it to the rest of the body. The left and right sides of the heart are separated by a wall of muscle called the septum. Altogether, these parts work to keep blood pumping continuously throughout the human body.

IN THE FLESH

The left ventricle is the largest and strongest chamber of the heart. It needs to be strong to pump blood throughout the body.

VALVES OF THE HEART

The heart has four **valves** that control blood flow. The tricuspid valve controls blood flow between the right atrium and right ventricle. The **pulmonary** valve allows blood to flow from the right ventricle out to the lungs to get oxygen. Oxygen-rich blood from the lungs passes from the left atrium into the left ventricle through the mitral valve. The aortic valve allows blood to pass from the left ventricle out to the rest of your body.

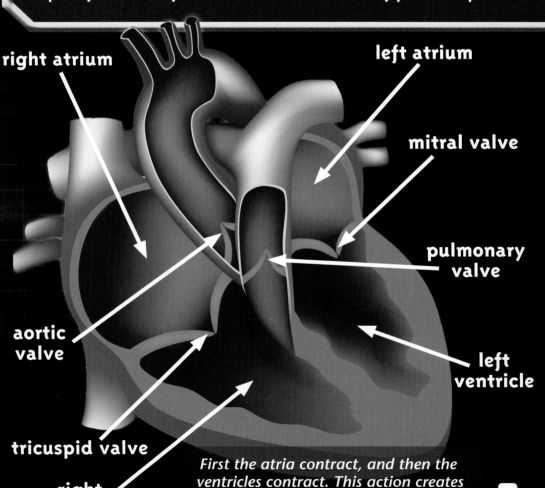

right atrium

left atrium

mitral valve

pulmonary valve

aortic valve

left ventricle

tricuspid valve

right ventricle

First the atria contract, and then the ventricles contract. This action creates the sound of your heart beating.

9

Blood Vessels

Blood circulates through hollow tubes called blood vessels. As the vessels extend farther and farther from the heart, they branch out into increasingly smaller tubes.

The human body has three kinds of blood vessels. Arteries, the strongest of the blood vessels, carry blood away from the heart. Except for the pulmonary arteries, arteries deliver oxygenated, or oxygen-rich, blood throughout the body. The aorta, which begins at the left ventricle, is the largest artery. It rises out of the top of the heart, turns downward, and extends just below the **diaphragm**. Carotid arteries travel up the neck and provide the brain with oxygenated blood. The femoral arteries are large blood vessels that run through the thighs.

IN THE FLESH

The pulmonary arteries carry blood from the heart to the lungs to get oxygen. They're the only arteries that carry deoxygenated blood, or blood from which oxygen has been removed.

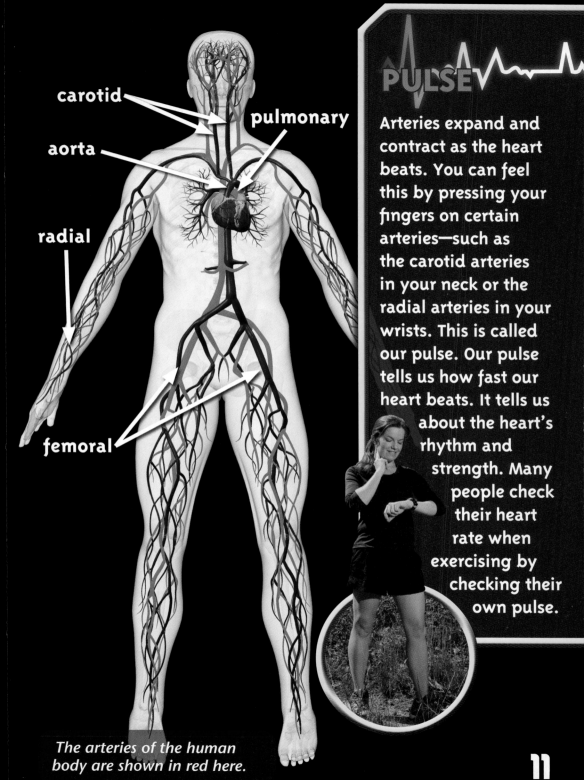

carotid

pulmonary

aorta

radial

femoral

PULSE

Arteries expand and contract as the heart beats. You can feel this by pressing your fingers on certain arteries—such as the carotid arteries in your neck or the radial arteries in your wrists. This is called our pulse. Our pulse tells us how fast our heart beats. It tells us about the heart's rhythm and strength. Many people check their heart rate when exercising by checking their own pulse.

The arteries of the human body are shown in red here.

Veins carry oxygen-poor blood from the tissues of the body back to the heart. They're thinner than arteries and not as strong. Since the veins carry the body's waste products, it's important that blood isn't allowed to flow backwards in them. To stop this from happening, veins have tiny valves to keep blood flowing toward the heart. The largest veins are the superior vena cava and inferior vena cava. These veins connect directly to the heart.

Capillaries connect the arteries to the veins. They're the smallest of the blood vessels; most are only one cell thick. Capillaries are so thin that oxygen and nutrients pass through their walls and into the surrounding tissues. Carbon dioxide passes from the tissues into the capillaries.

IN THE FLESH

The pulmonary veins carry blood from the lungs to the heart. They're the only veins that carry oxygenated blood.

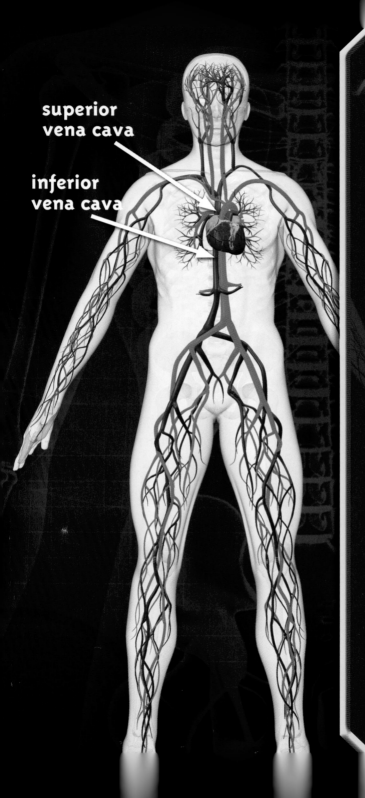

superior
vena cava

inferior
vena cava

THREE LAYERS

Arteries and veins have three layers. The outside layer supports the vessel by connecting it to surrounding tissues. This holds the vessel in place. The middle layer is muscle, which works with the heart to keep blood flowing. It's usually the thickest layer. The inner layer is very thin. It's the layer that's in contact with the blood.

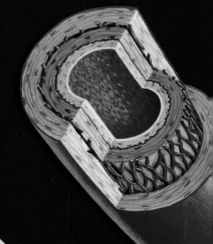

Types of Circulation

Two kinds of circulation occur within the circulatory system. Pulmonary circulation involves the movement of deoxygenated blood from the heart to the lungs and oxygenated blood from the lungs to the heart. Blood reaches the lungs through the pulmonary arteries. Capillaries in the lungs exchange carbon dioxide for oxygen, and the blood travels back to the heart through the pulmonary veins.

Systemic circulation involves the movement of oxygenated blood from the heart to the body and deoxygenated blood from the body back to the heart. Blood leaves the heart through the aorta, which branches out into increasingly smaller arteries. After passing through the capillaries and releasing its oxygen, the deoxygenated blood returns to the heart through the veins.

IN THE FLESH

The muscle layer in arteries is very strong to help keep blood pumping. The interior layer is very smooth. This allows blood to flow more quickly.

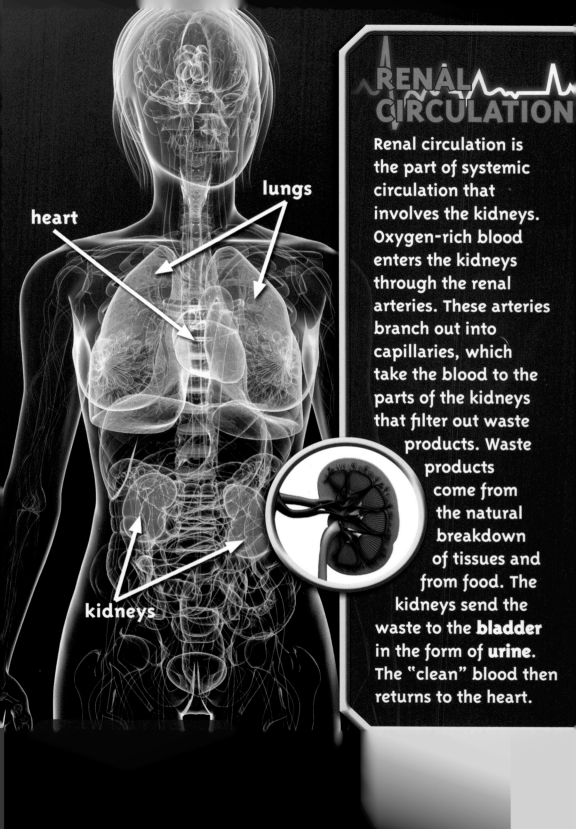

heart

lungs

kidneys

Renal circulation is the part of systemic circulation that involves the kidneys. Oxygen-rich blood enters the kidneys through the renal arteries. These arteries branch out into capillaries, which take the blood to the parts of the kidneys that filter out waste products. Waste products come from the natural breakdown of tissues and from food. The kidneys send the waste to the **bladder** in the form of **urine**. The "clean" blood then returns to the heart.

In the Blood

People can't live without blood. It brings oxygen and nutrients to every cell in the body. It also carries waste products away. Blood helps keep us warm when it's cold, and it helps cool us off when it's hot.

Blood is made up of two parts: cells and a clear, yellowish liquid called plasma. The average adult has approximately 5.3 quarts (5 l) of blood. About 55 percent of that is plasma. About 90 percent of plasma is water. The other 10 percent is made up of waste products and nutrients we need for life. This includes proteins—nutrients our bodies need to build, maintain, and replace tissues. It also includes hormones, which are chemicals that affect the way our bodies function.

IN THE FLESH

Blood makes up 7 to 8 percent of a person's body weight.

red blood cell

white blood cell

lymph node

WHAT IS LYMPH?

When blood enters capillaries, some plasma passes into the surrounding tissues. It carries nutrients to cells and removes wastes. Most of the plasma reenters the circulatory system, but a small portion remains behind. This clear liquid is called lymph. Lymph travels toward the neck through the vessels that make up the lymphatic system.
Wastes in lymph are filtered out by small lumps of tissue called nodes. Then, the lymph reenters the circulatory system as plasma.

The cells in our blood include red blood cells, white blood cells, and platelets. Each cell has a different function.

platelet

Blood cells are made by **bone marrow**. In children, blood cells are made in the marrow of most bones. In adults, blood cells are produced in the marrow of the spine, breastbone, ribs, pelvis, upper arms, and upper legs.

Red blood cells (RBCs) carry oxygen from the lungs to the rest of the body. RBCs are round, flat disks with a biconcave shape. This means the

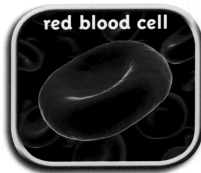

red blood cell

surfaces on both sides of a cell curve inward. As blood passes through the lungs, oxygen attaches itself to a molecule in RBCs called hemoglobin. Oxygen-rich blood is red, and oxygen-poor blood is bluish-purple. RBCs wear out after about 120 days. They're replaced by new cells. Old RBCs are removed from the body by the **liver** and **spleen**.

IN THE FLESH

Blood loss can occur due to an injury or during surgery. This blood can be replaced with another person's blood. The process of replacing blood is call a transfusion.

BLOOD TYPE

If you've ever given blood, you know that blood comes in different "types." The different types are based on the presence or absence of proteins on the surface of RBCs. These proteins are called A and B. When someone is **donating** their blood to someone else, it's very important to know what type of blood both people have or problems can occur.

blood type	protein	blood donations
A	A	can be donated to As and ABs
B	B	can be donated to Bs and ABs
AB	both A and B	can be donated only to ABs
O	neither A nor B	can be donated to anyone

White blood cells (WBCs) help fight illnesses in the body. Everyone gets infections from time to time. An infection happens when germs enter the body and then increase in number. Germs are tiny living things that can only be seen under a microscope. The most common types of germs are bacteria. Some kinds of bacteria make people sick. WBCs help fight "bad" bacteria and other germs that enter the body.

There are five major types of WBCs. Each has a different job. Some only go after a specific kind of germ. They surround the germs and "eat" them. Other WBCs use proteins called antibodies to attack germs. In people with **allergies**, WBCs attack normally harmless substances, such as dust, pollen, and mold.

IN THE FLESH

There are fewer white blood cells in the bloodstream than red blood cells. However, white blood cell production increases when germs appear.

PLATELETS AND CLOTTING

When blood vessels are damaged or cut, oval cells called platelets rush to the injury. The platelets branch out and fit together like puzzle pieces to seal the wound. These tiny cells use a protein to help them stick together. The clump that forms is called a clot. It forms a plug that keeps blood inside the vessels and germs outside. Platelets form scabs over cuts on the skin.

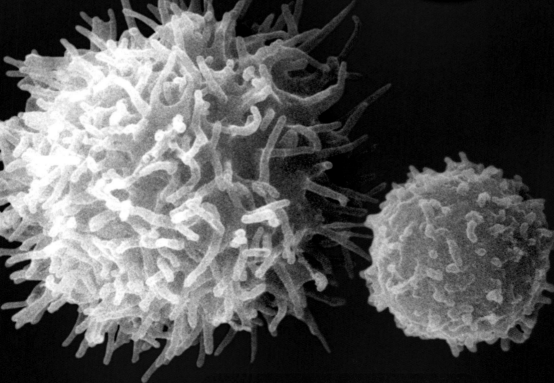

platelets

Depending on the kind, WBCs live from a few days to a few weeks.

Chemical Messengers

In addition to oxygen, nutrients, and waste, the circulatory system also transports chemicals known as hormones. In the human body, organs called glands make hormones and secrete, or release, them into the bloodstream. Hormones are sometimes called "chemical messengers" because

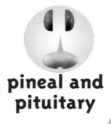

pineal and pituitary

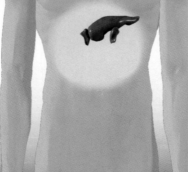

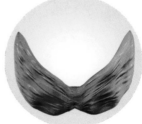

thyroid

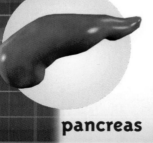

pancreas

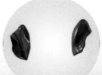

adrenals

Shown here are some of the major glands of the human body.

they give organs information about how to function. This happens all the time in the human body. Hormones wouldn't be able to get where they need to go without the circulatory system.

There are numerous glands in the human body. The heart itself sometimes acts as a gland. Under certain conditions, it secretes a hormone that helps regulate blood flow and kidney function. When secreted, this hormone tells the kidneys to release larger-than-normal amounts of salt in the urine. This, in turn, removes excess water from the blood.

FIGHT OR FLIGHT?

The "fight or flight response" is the human body's inborn ability to prepare for a fight or run away. The brain first sends messages to several parts of the body, including glands. Adrenaline from the adrenal glands tells the heart to beat faster. It causes the arteries to grow narrower and the veins wider. This increases blood flow throughout the body. The pituitary gland releases endorphins—natural painkillers—into the bloodstream.

IN THE FLESH

Together, all the glands in the human body make up the endocrine system. The word "endocrine" comes from the Greek words for "inside" and "secrete."

Diseases and Disorders

There are many diseases and disorders related to the circulatory system. Some affect the heart, some affect the blood vessels, and some affect the blood.

"Heart disease" is a general term for any disease that affects the blood vessels and heart. It's the number one cause of death in the United States. The most common form is coronary artery disease. Fatty material builds up on artery walls, causing them to become narrow and "hardened." Blood flow to the heart is reduced. This can cause chest pain and heart attack. A heart attack can result in permanent heart damage or death. Other common forms of heart disease include an uneven heartbeat and heart failure, which occurs when the heart can't pump enough blood throughout the body.

IN THE FLESH

Blood pressure is a measurement of the force of blood pumping through the arteries. Hypertension (high blood pressure) and hypotension (low blood pressure) are signs of heart disease.

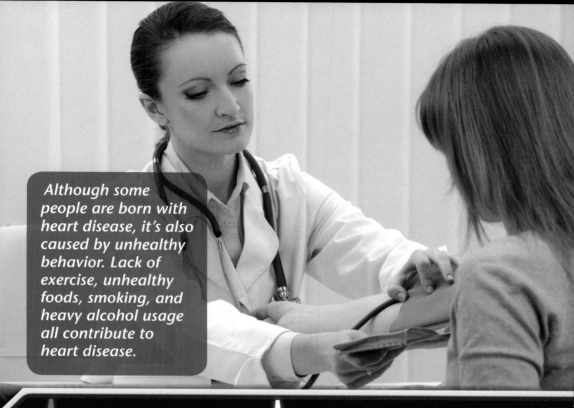

Although some people are born with heart disease, it's also caused by unhealthy behavior. Lack of exercise, unhealthy foods, smoking, and heavy alcohol usage all contribute to heart disease.

WHAT'S A STENT?

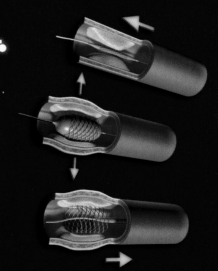

Patients with coronary artery disease are benefiting from an amazing yet simple medical device. A stent is a small, wire-mesh tube designed to widen blocked arteries and restore normal blood flow. A balloon is placed inside the stent. Doctors make a small cut in an arm or leg artery and then slide the stent along the artery to the blockage. The balloon is filled with air, which causes the stent—as well as the artery—to open up.

Many illnesses affect the blood. Some are passed from parent to child, but others can happen to anyone. Anemia is a condition in which the blood doesn't have enough RBCs or the RBCs don't have enough hemoglobin. People with anemia have oxygen-poor blood and often feel tired. Most cases are mild, but severe cases can damage the body's organs and lead to death.

People with hemophilia, a rare disorder, have blood that doesn't clot properly. They bleed longer than other people and can suffer from internal bleeding. Most cases of hemophilia are passed from parent to child.

A pulmonary embolism is a sudden blockage in a lung artery. It's usually caused by a blood clot that travels from a vein in a leg to the lungs. It can be life threatening if not treated immediately.

IN THE FLESH

Anything that enters the bloodstream is carried throughout the human body. This is how many illnesses make us sick. Pests, such as mosquitoes and rats, can pass deadly illnesses to humans with a single bite.

The misshapen RBC at the bottom of the page is the result of a disease called sickle cell anemia. It's caused by abnormal hemoglobin.

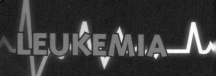

LEUKEMIA

Leukemia is a **cancer** that affects the bone marrow and blood. Bone marrow in people with leukemia produces a large number of WBCs that don't act like normal cells. In time, these abnormal WBCs crowd out healthy cells in the bloodstream, lymph nodes, liver, and spleen. Leukemia causes anemia, bleeding, and infections. Some forms of leukemia can be cured, some can be controlled, and others are deadly.

Have a Healthy Heart

A regular exercise routine strengthens the circulatory system and improves blood flow. This helps the human body use oxygen better. Exercise also helps fight hypertension.

Eating too many fatty and sugary foods leads to hypertension and coronary artery disease. Too much salt can also lead to hypertension. A diet high in fruits, vegetables, whole grains, and low-fat proteins will help keep your heart healthy.

Among many other illnesses smoking causes, it can increase the buildup of fat in the arteries. It can also make it difficult to breathe and reduce the amount of oxygenated blood that travels throughout the body. The use of legal and illegal drugs can dangerously speed up or slow down the heart. A healthy lifestyle helps keep the circulatory system running strong!

The Circulatory System

- If you could remove the blood vessels from a person's body and lay them out in a straight line, they would be over 60,000 miles (96,500 km) long!

- Blood takes about 20 seconds to make one trip throughout the circulatory system.

- An adult woman's heart weighs about 8 ounces (227 g).

- An adult man's heart weighs about 10 ounces (283 g).

- Blood pressure is measured using two numbers. The higher number is measured when the heart beats. The lower number is measured between beats.

- A drop of blood contains millions of RBCs.

  - A drop of blood can have between 7,000 and 25,000 WBCs. Someone with leukemia might have 50,000 WBCs in a single drop of blood.

  - Capillaries enlarge when we exercise to release heat and keep our body temperature down. This is why our skin looks red and flushed.

Glossary

allergy: a sensitivity to normally harmless things in the environment, such as dust, pollen, or mold

arthropod: an animal that lacks a backbone and has a skeleton on the outside of its body, such as an insect, spider, shrimp, or crab

bladder: an expandable organ that stores liquid waste until it can be removed from the body

bone marrow: soft matter inside bones where blood cells are made

cancer: a disease caused by the uncontrolled growth of cells in the body

diaphragm: a thin, curved muscle below the lungs

donate: to give something, such as blood, to others who need it

liver: an organ that stores and cleans blood

mollusk: an animal that lacks a backbone and has a soft body, such as a snail, clam, or octopus

nutrient: something a living thing needs to grow and stay alive

pulmonary: relating to or affecting the lungs

spleen: an organ that destroys old blood cells and stores blood

urine: yellowish liquid secreted by the kidneys that contains waste products

valve: something that controls the movement of liquids or gases through tubes or vessels

For More Information

BOOKS

Parker, Steve. *Circulatory System*. Mankato, MN: New Forest Press, 2010.

Romanek, Trudee. *Squirt! The Most Interesting Book You'll Ever Read About Blood*. Toronto, ON, Canada: Kids Can Press, 2006.

Taylor-Butler, Christine. *The Circulatory System*. New York, NY: Children's Press, 2008.

WEBSITES

American Heart Association
www.heart.org
Learn more about heart disease and how you can increase your chances of living a long, healthy life.

The Immune Platoon
www.bam.gov/sub_diseases/diseases_immuneplatoon.html
Watch this fun, animated presentation to learn more about white blood cells and how they help protect your body from germs and infections.

Your Heart and Circulatory System
kidshealth.org/kid/htbw/heart.html
Read more about the circulatory system.

Index